THE COMPLETE PLANT BASED DIET COOKBOOK FOR WOMAN OVER 50

Amazing and Mouth-watering Recipes for busy people. How to Kick-start your Weight loss Journey with amazing dishes.

Ursa Males

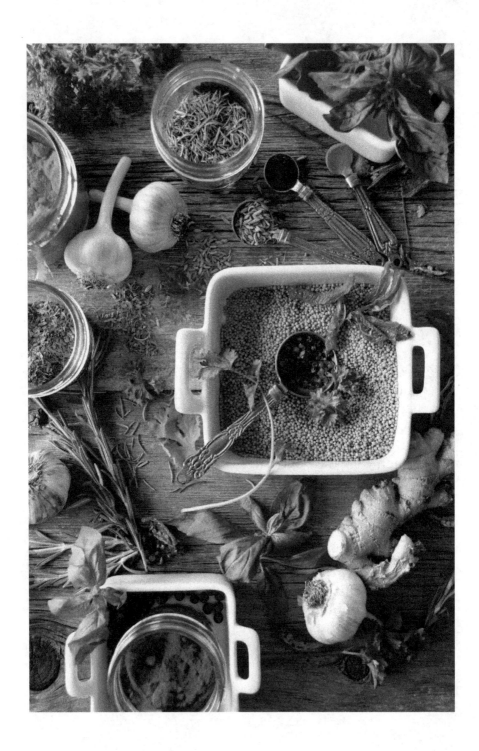

TABLE OF CONTENTS

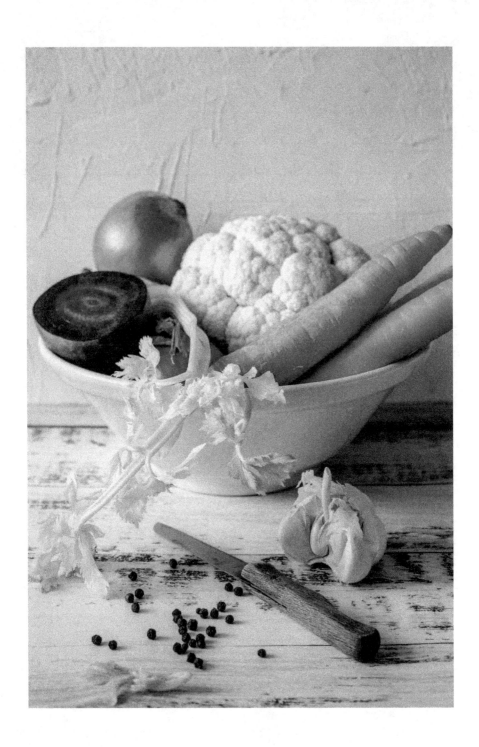

BREAKFAST

1. Fruity Granola

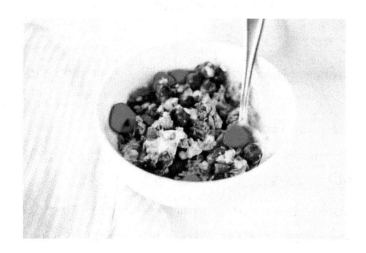

Preparation time: 15 minutes

Cooking time: 45 minutes

Servings: 5 cups

Ingredients:

- 2 cups rolled oats
- ¾ cup whole-grain flour
- 1 tablespoon ground cinnamon
- 1 teaspoon ground ginger (optional)
- ½ cup sunflower seeds, or walnuts, chopped
- ½ cup almonds, chopped
- ½ cup pumpkin seeds

- ½ cup unsweetened shredded coconut
- 1¼ cups pure fruit juice (cranberry, apple, or something similar)
- ½ cup raisins, or dried cranberries
- ½ cup goji berries (optional)

Directions:

1. Preheat the oven to 350°F. Mix the oats, flour, cinnamon, ginger, sunflower seeds, almonds, pumpkin seeds, and coconut in a large bowl.
2. Sprinkle the juice over the batter, then mix until it's just moistened.
3. Spread the granola on a large baking sheet (the more spread out it is, the better), and put it in the oven. After about 15 minutes, use a spatula to turn the granola so that the middle gets dried out.
4. Let the granola bake until it's as crunchy as you want it, about 30 minutes more. Remove the granola and stir in the raisins and goji berries (if using). Serve.

Nutrition: Calories: 398 Fat: 25g Carbs: 39g Protein: 11g

2. <u>Roasted Veg with Creamy Avocado Dip</u>

Preparation time: 10 minutes

Cooking time: 30 minutes

Servings: 2

Ingredients:

- For the avocado dip:
- 1 avocado
- 1 tablespoon apple cider vinegar
- ¼ to ½ cup of water
- 2 tablespoons nutritional yeast
- 1 teaspoon dried dill/1 tablespoon fresh dill
- Pinch sea salt
- For the roasted veg:
- 1 small sweet potato, peeled and cubed
- 2 small beets, peeled and cubed
- 2 small carrots, peeled and cubed
- 1 teaspoon of sea salt
- 1 teaspoon dried oregano
- ¼ teaspoon cayenne pepper
- Pinch freshly ground black pepper

Directions:

1. To make the avocado dip:
2. In a blender, purée the avocado with the other dip ingredients, using just enough water to get a smooth, creamy texture.
3. Alternatively, you can mash the avocado thoroughly in a large bowl and then stir in the rest of the dip ingredients.
4. To make the roasted veg:
5. Preheat the oven to 350°F. Put the sweet potato, beets, and carrots in a large pot with a small amount of water, and bring to a boil over high heat.
6. Boil for 15 minutes, until they're just barely soft, then drain. Sprinkle the salt, oregano, cayenne, and pepper over them and stir gently to combine. (Use more or less cayenne depending on your taste.)
7. Spread the vegetables on a large baking sheet and roast them in the oven for 10 to 15 minutes until they've browned around the edges. Serve the veg with the avocado dip on the side.

Nutrition: Calories: 335 Fat: 12g Carbs: 51g Protein: 11g

3. Lovely Baby Potatoes

Preparation Time: 10 minutes

Cooking Time: 35 minutes

Servings: 4

Ingredients:

- 2 pounds new yellow potatoes, scrubbed and cut into wedges
- 2 tablespoons extra virgin olive oil
- 2 teaspoons fresh rosemary, chopped
- 1 teaspoon garlic powder
- ½ teaspoon freshly ground black pepper and sunflower seeds

Directions:

1. Preheat your oven to 400 degrees Fahrenheit. Line baking sheet with aluminum foil and set aside. Take a large bowl and add potatoes, olive oil, garlic, rosemary, sea sunflower seeds, and pepper.
2. Spread potatoes in a single layer on a baking sheet and bake for 35 minutes.

3. Serve and enjoy!

Nutrition: Calories: 225 Fat: 7g Carbohydrates: 37g Protein: 5g

4. <u>Apple Porridge</u>

Preparation Time: 10 minutes

Cooking Time: 5 minutes

Servings: 2

Ingredients:

- 1 large apple, peeled, cored, and grated
- 1 cup unsweetened almond milk
- 1 ½ tablespoon of sunflower seeds
- 1/8 cup of fresh blueberries
- ¼ teaspoon of fresh vanilla bean extract

Directions:

1. Take a large pan and add sunflower seeds, vanilla extract, almond milk, apples, and stir. Place it over medium-low heat.
2. Cook for 5 minutes, making sure to keep stirring the mixture. Transfer to a serving bowl. Serve and enjoy!

Nutrition: Calories: 123 Fat: 1.3g Carbohydrates: 23g Protein: 4g

5. Simple Granola Platter

Preparation time: 5 minutes

Cooking time: 25 minutes

Servings: 4

Ingredients:

- 1-ounce porridge oats
- 2 teaspoons of maple syrup
- Cooking spray as needed
- 4 medium bananas
- 5-ounce fresh fruit salad, such as strawberries, blueberries, and raspberries
- ¼ ounce pumpkin seeds
- ¼ ounce sunflower seeds
- ¼ ounce dry Chia seeds
- ¼ ounce desiccated coconut

Directions:

1. Preheat your oven to 300 degrees Fahrenheit. Prepare a baking tray then line it with baking paper. Take a large bowl and add oats, maple syrup, and seeds.
2. Spread mix on a baking tray. Spray coconut oil on top and bake for 20 minutes, making sure to keep stirring it from time to time.

3. Sprinkle coconut after the first 15 minutes. Remove from oven and let it cool. Take a bowl and layer sliced bananas. Spread the cooled granola mix on top and serve with a topping of berries. Enjoy!

Nutrition: Calories: 446 Fat: 29g Carbohydrates: 37g Protein: 13g

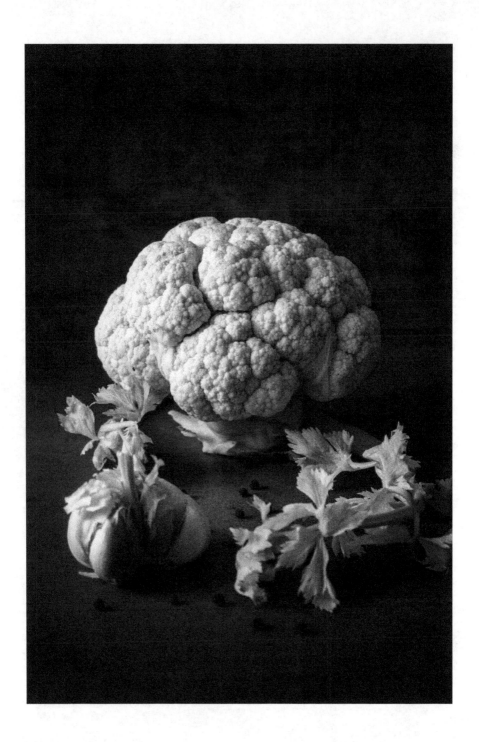

LUNCH

6. Avocado and Cauliflower Hummus

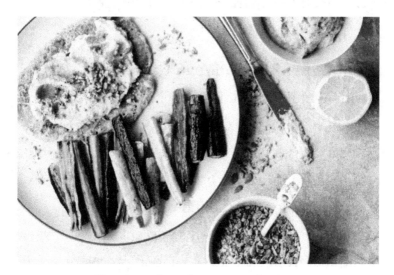

Preparation time: 45 minutes

Cooking time: 20-25 minutes

Servings: 2

Ingredients:

- 1 medium cauliflower (stem removed and chopped)
- 1 large Hass avocado (peeled, pitted, and chopped)
- ¼ cup extra virgin olive oil
- 2 garlic cloves
- ½ tbsp. lemon juice
- ½ tsp. onion powder

- Sea salt
- ground black pepper
- 2 large carrots (peeled & cut into fries, or use store-bought raw carrot fries)
- Optional: ¼ cup fresh cilantro (chopped)

Directions:

1. Warm oven to 450°F/220°C, and line a baking tray with aluminum foil. Put the chopped cauliflower on the baking tray and drizzle with 2 tablespoons of olive oil.
2. Roast the chopped cauliflower in the oven for 20-25 minutes, until lightly brown. Remove the tray from the oven and allow the cauliflower to cool down.
3. Add all the ingredients—except the carrots and optional fresh cilantro—to a food processor or blender, and blend them into a smooth hummus.
4. Transfer the hummus to a medium-sized bowl, cover, and put it in the fridge for at least 30 minutes.
5. Take the hummus out of the fridge and, if desired, top it with the optional chopped cilantro and more salt and pepper to taste; serve with the carrot fries, and enjoy!

Nutrition: Calories: 416 Carbs: 8.4 g. Fat: 40.3 g. Protein: 3.3 g.

7. Raw Zoodles with Avocado 'N Nuts

Preparation time: 15 minutes

Cooking time: 0 minutes

Servings: 2

Ingredients:

- 1 medium zucchini (spiralized into zoodles or sliced into skinny slices)
- 1½ cups basil
- 1/3 cup water
- 5 tbsp. pine nuts
- 2 tbsp. lemon juice
- 1 medium avocado (peeled, pitted, and sliced)
- Optional: 2 tbsp. olive oil
- 6 yellow cherry tomatoes (halved)
- Optional: 6 red cherry tomatoes (halved)
- Sea salt and black pepper to taste

Directions:

1. Add the basil, water, nuts, lemon juice, avocado slices, optional olive oil (if desired), salt, and pepper to a blender. Blend the ingredients into a smooth mixture. Add more salt plus pepper to taste and blend again.
2. Divide the sauce and the zucchini noodles between two medium-sized bowls for serving, and combine in each.

3. Top the mixtures with the halved yellow cherry tomatoes and the optional red cherry tomatoes (if desired); serve and enjoy!

4. Alternatively, store the zoodles in the fridge using an airtight container and consume them within 2 days.

Nutrition: Calories: 317 Carbs: 7.4 g. Fat: 28.1 g. Protein: 7.2 g.

8. Cauliflower Sushi

Preparation time: 15 minutes

Cooking time: 0 minutes

Servings: 4

Ingredients:

- Sushi Base:
- 6 cups cauliflower florets (or 15-oz. pack cauliflower rice)
- ½ cup vegan cheese
- 1 medium spring onion (diced)
- 4 nori sheets
- Sea salt and pepper to taste
- 1 tbsp. rice vinegar or sushi vinegar
- Optional: 1 medium garlic clove (minced)
- Filling:
- 1 medium Hass avocado (peeled, sliced)
- ½ medium cucumber (skinned, sliced)
- 4 asparagus spears
- Optional: a handful of enoki mushrooms

Directions:

1. Put the cauliflower florets in your food processor or blender. Pulse the florets into a rice-like substance.

When using readymade cauliflower rice, add this to the blender.

2. Add the vegan cheese, spring onions, and vinegar to the food processor or blender. Top these ingredients with salt and pepper to taste, and pulse everything into a chunky mixture.

3. Taste, then put more vinegar, salt, or pepper to taste. Add the optional minced garlic clove to the blender and pulse again for a few seconds.

4. Layout the nori sheets and spread the cauliflower rice mixture out evenly between the sheets. Make sure to leave at least 2 inches of the top and bottom edges empty.

5. Place one or more combinations of multiple filling ingredients along the center of the spread-out rice mixture. Experiment with different ingredients per nori sheet for the best flavor.

6. Roll up each nori sheet tightly. Either serve the sushi as a nori roll or slice each roll up into sushi pieces.

7. Serve right away with a small amount of wasabi, pickled ginger, and soy sauce!

Nutrition: Calories: 189 Carbs: 7.6 g. Fat: 14.4 g. Protein: 6.1 g.

9. <u>Keto Curry Almond Bread</u>

Preparation time: 15 minutes

Cooking time: 0 minutes

Servings: 2

Ingredients:

- ½ cup almond flour (or coconut flour)
- ¼ cup almond milk
- ¼ cup ground flaxseed
- 2 tbsp. coconut oil
- 2 tbsp red curry paste
- ½ tsp salt
- ½ tsp cane sugar (or stevia powder)
- 2 kaffir lime leaves (chopped)
- 2 tsp. dried ginger (or fresh, minced)
- Optional: ¼ cup of water
- Optional: 4 tbsp. coconut flakes

Directions:

1. Line a baking sheet with parchment paper. Mix the almond milk with the sugar, salt, and ground flaxseeds in a medium bowl. Stir well and let it sit for 10 minutes.
2. Add the flour, kaffir lime leaves, and ginger to the bowl. Incorporate all ingredients using your hands or an

electric mixer. Add some of the optional water to make the mixing easier.

3. Split the dough into two pieces, then flatten these out onto the baking sheet. Grease both sides of the dough with coconut oil and apply a tablespoon of red curry paste on each flattened bread's top side.

4. Allow the pieces of bread to rest for an hour at room temperature. Warm oven to 400°F / 200°C. Bake the bread for about 15 minutes, until golden brown on top.

5. Top the bread with the optional coconut flakes. Serve and enjoy!

Nutrition: Calories: 372 Carbs: 5.1 g. Fat: 34.7 g. Protein: 8.3 g.

10. **Shio Koji Karaage Tofu**

Preparation time: 15 minutes

Cooking time: 10 minutes

Servings: 4

Ingredients:

- Extra light olive oil (for deep-frying)
- 1 12-oz. pack extra firm tofu (drained, cubed)
- 4 tbsp. Hikari Shio Koji
- 1 tsp. fresh ginger (finely chopped)
- 1 garlic clove (minced)
- 2 tsp. soy sauce
- ½ cup almond flour
- Optional: lemon wedges

Directions:

1. Combine the tofu cubes with the Hikari Shio Koji, ginger, garlic, and soy sauce in a large bowl or Ziploc bag.

2. Use your hands to make sure the tofu is evenly coated. Cover the bowl or close the Ziploc bag and put it in the fridge. Marinate the tofu for at least 30 minutes up to a maximum of 1 day.

3. Heat a pot with enough olive oil to deep fry the tofu cubes. The ideal temperature for the oil is 325°F /160°F.

4. Take the tofu cubes out of the fridge and cover the cubes with almond flour. It can be done in a bowl or Ziploc bag. Use your hands to coat all tofu cubes with flour evenly.

5. Drop the coated cubes gently into the pot and fry until they're lightly browned. When the tofu cubes are ready, transfer them to a plate lined with paper towels to drain the excess oil.

6. Serve the shio koji karaage tofu, garnished with the optional lemon wedges if desired, and enjoy!

Nutrition: Calories: 355 Carbs: 4.9 g. Fat: 32 g. Protein: 11.3 g.

11. <u>Mushrooms Sandwich</u>

Preparation time: 10 minutes

Cooking time: 5 minutes

Servings: 4

Ingredients:

- 8 cherry tomatoes, halved
- 2 ounces of baby spinach
- 20 ounces of oyster mushrooms
- 2/3 teaspoon salt
- 1/3 teaspoon ground black pepper
- 2 tablespoons olive oil
- 4 tablespoons of barbecue sauce
- 8 slices of bread, toasted

Directions:

1. Take a griddle pan, place it over medium-high heat, grease it with oil and let it preheat.
2. Cut mushroom into thin strips, add to the hot griddle pan, drizzle with oil and cook for 5 minutes until done.
3. Transfer grilled mushrooms into a medium bowl, season with salt and black pepper, add barbecue sauce and toss until mixed.

4. Spread prepared mushroom mixture evenly on four bread slices, top with spinach and cherry tomatoes, then cover with the other four slices and serve.

Nutrition: Cal 350 Fat 11 g Carbohydrates 46 g Protein 12.1 g

12. Rainbow Taco Boats

Preparation time: 10 minutes

Cooking time: 0 minutes

Servings: 4

Ingredients:

- 1 head romaine lettuce, destemmed
- For the Filling:
- 1/2 cup alfalfa sprouts
- 1 medium avocado, peeled, pitted, cubed
- 1 cup shredded carrots
- 1 cup halved cherry tomatoes
- 3/4 cup sliced red cabbage
- 1/2 cup sprouted hummus dip
- 1 tablespoon hemp seeds
- For the Sauce:
- 1 tablespoon maple syrup
- 1/3 cup tahini
- 1/8 teaspoon sea salt
- 2 tablespoons lemon juice
- 3 tablespoons water

Directions:

1. Prepare the sauce and for this, take a medium bowl, add all the ingredients in it and whisk until well combined.
2. Assemble the boats, arrange lettuce leaves in twelve portions, top each with hummus and the remaining ingredients for the filling. Serve with prepared sauce.

Nutrition: Cal 314 Fat 23.6 g Carbohydrates 23.2 g Protein 8 g

13. **Eggplant Sandwich**

Preparation time: 10 minutes

Cooking time: 25 minutes

Servings: 4

Ingredients:

- For the Sandwich:
- 2 ciabatta buns
- 1 medium eggplant, peeled, sliced, soaked in salted water
- 1 medium tomato, sliced
- 1/2 of a medium cucumber, sliced
- 1/2 cup arugula
- 4 tablespoons mayo
- For the Marinade:
- 1 teaspoon agave syrup
- 1/4 teaspoon salt
- 1/4 teaspoon ground black pepper
- 1 teaspoon smoked paprika
- 1 tablespoon soy sauce
- 1 tablespoon olive oil

Directions:

1. Switch on the oven, then set it to 350 degrees F and let it preheat. Prepare the marinade and for this, take a

small bowl, place all the ingredients in it and whisk until combined.

2. Drain the eggplant slices, pat dry with a kitchen towel, brush with prepared marinade, arrange them on a baking sheet and then bake for 20 minutes until done.

3. Assemble the sandwich and for this, slice the bread in half lengthwise, then spread mayonnaise in the bottom half of the bun and top with baked eggplant slices, tomato, and cucumber slices, and sprinkle with salt and black pepper.

4. Top with arugula leaves, cover with the top half of the bun and then cover with aluminum foil.

5. Preheat the grill over a medium-high heat setting, and when hot, place prepared sandwiches and grill for 3 to 5 minutes until toasted. Cut each sandwich through the foil into half and serve.

Nutrition: Cal 688 Fat 15 g Carbohydrates 118 g Protein 21 g

Lentil, Cauliflower and Grape Salad

14. **<u>Preparation time: 10 minutes</u>**

Cooking time: 25 minutes

Servings: 4

Ingredients:

For the Cauliflower:

- 1 medium head of cauliflower, sliced into florets
- 1/4 teaspoon sea salt
- 1 1/2 tablespoons curry powder
- 1 1/2 tablespoons melted coconut oil
- For the Tahini Dressing:
- 2 tablespoons tahini
- 1/8 teaspoon salt
- 1 3/4 teaspoon ground black pepper
- 4 1/2 tablespoons green curry paste
- 1 tablespoon maple syrup
- 2 tablespoons lemon juice
- 2 tablespoons water
- For the Salad:
- 1 cup cooked lentils
- 4 tablespoons chopped cilantro
- 1 cup red grapes, halved
- 6 cups mixed greens

Directions:

1. Switch on the oven, then set it to 400 degrees F and let it preheat. Prepare the cauliflower and for this, take a medium bowl, place cauliflower florets in it, drizzle with oil, season with salt and curry powder, toss until mixed.

2. Take a baking sheet, line it with a parchment sheet, spread cauliflower florets in it, and then bake for 25 minutes until tender and nicely golden brown.

3. Meanwhile, prepare the tahini dressing, take a medium bowl, place all of its ingredients, and whisk until combined, set aside until required.

4. Assemble the salad and for this, take a large salad bowl, add roasted cauliflower florets, lentils, grapes, and mixed greens, drizzle with prepared tahini dressing and toss until well combined. Serve straight away.

Nutrition: Cal 420 Fat 14 g Carbohydrates 37.6 g Protein 10.8 g

15. Loaded Kale Salad

Preparation time: 10 minutes

Cooking time: 30 minutes

Servings: 4

Ingredients:

- 1 ½ cup cooked quinoa
- For the Vegetables:
- 1 whole beet, peeled, sliced
- 4 large carrots, peeled, chopped
- 1/2 teaspoon curry powder
- 1/8 teaspoon sea salt
- 2 tablespoons melted coconut oil
- For the Dressing:
- ¼ teaspoon of sea salt
- 2 tablespoons maple syrup
- 3 tablespoons lemon juice
- 1/3 cup tahini
- 1/4 cup water
- For the Salad:
- 1/2 cup sprouts
- 1 medium avocado, peeled, pitted, cubed
- 1/2 cup chopped cherry tomatoes

- 8 cups chopped kale
- 1/4 cup hemp seeds

Directions:

1. Switch on the oven, then set it to 375 degrees F and let it preheat. Take a baking sheet, place beets and carrots on it, drizzle with oil, season with curry powder and salt, toss until coated, and then bake for 30 minutes until tender and golden brown.
2. Meanwhile, prepare the dressing and for this, take a small bowl, place all the ingredients in it and whisk until well combined, set aside until required.
3. Assemble the salad and for this, take a large salad bowl, place kale leaves in it, add remaining ingredients for the salad along with roasted vegetables, drizzle with prepared dressing and toss until combined. Serve straight away.

Nutrition: Cal 472 Fat 22.8 g Carbohydrates 58.7 g Protein 14.6 g

DINNER

16. <u>Smoky Red Beans and Rice</u>

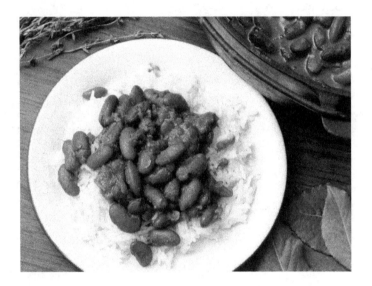

Preparation Time: 15 minutes

Cooking Time: 6 minutes

Servings: 6

Ingredients:

- 30 ounces of cooked red beans
- 1 cup of brown rice, uncooked
- 1 cup of chopped green pepper
- 1 cup of chopped celery
- 1 cup of chopped white onion
- 1 1/2 teaspoon of minced garlic

- 1/2 teaspoon of salt
- 1/4 teaspoon of cayenne pepper
- 1 teaspoon of smoked paprika
- 2 teaspoons of dried thyme
- 1 bay leaf
- 2 1/3 cups of vegetable broth

Directions:

1. Using a 6-quarts slow cooker, place all the ingredients except for the rice, salt, and cayenne pepper. Stir until it mixes properly and then cover the top.
2. Plug in the slow cooker, adjust the cooking time to 4 hours, and steam on a low heat setting.
3. Then pour in and stir the rice, salt, cayenne pepper and continue cooking for an additional 2 hours at a high heat setting. Serve straight away.

Nutrition: Calories: 791 Protein: 3.25 g Fat: 86.45 g Carbohydrates: 9.67 g

17.   Spicy Black-Eyed Peas

Preparation Time: 12 minutes

Cooking Time: 8 hours and 8 minutes

Servings: 8

Ingredients:

- 32-ounce black-eyed peas, uncooked
- 1 cup of chopped orange bell pepper
- 1 cup of chopped celery
- 8-ounce of chipotle peppers, chopped
- 1 cup of chopped carrot
- 1 cup of chopped white onion
- 1 teaspoon of minced garlic
- 3/4 teaspoon of salt
- 1/2 teaspoon of ground black pepper
- 2 teaspoons of liquid smoke flavoring
- 2 teaspoons of ground cumin
- 1 tablespoon of adobo sauce
- 2 tablespoons of olive oil
- 1 tablespoon of apple cider vinegar
- 4 cups of vegetable broth

Directions:

1. Place a medium-sized non-stick skillet pan over an average temperature of heat; add the bell peppers, carrot, onion, garlic, oil, and vinegar.

2. Stir until it mixes properly and let it cook for 5 to 8 minutes or until it gets translucent.

3. Transfer this mixture to a 6-quarts slow cooker and add the peas, chipotle pepper, adobo sauce, and the vegetable broth. Stir until mixed properly and cover the top.

4. Plug in the slow cooker, adjust the cooking time to 8 hours, and let it cook on the low heat setting or until peas are soft. Serve right away.

Nutrition: Calories: 1071 Protein: 5.3 g Fat: 113.65 g Carbohydrates: 18.51 g

18. Creamy Artichoke Soup

Preparation Time: 5 minutes

Cooking Time: 40 minutes

Servings: 4

Ingredients:

- 1 can artichoke hearts, drained
- 3 cups vegetable broth
- 2 tbsp. lemon juice
- 1 small onion, finely cut
- 2 cloves garlic, crushed
- 3 tbsp. olive oil
- 2 tbsp. flour
- ½ cup vegan cream

Directions:

1. Gently sauté the onion and garlic in some olive oil. Add the flour, whisking constantly, and then add the hot vegetable broth slowly, while still whisking. Cook for about 5 minutes.
2. Blend the artichoke, lemon juice, salt, and pepper until smooth. Add the puree to the broth mix, stir well, and then stir in the cream.

3. Cook until heated through. Garnish with a swirl of vegan cream or a sliver of artichoke.

Nutrition: Calories: 1622 Protein: 4.45 g Fat: 181.08 g Carbohydrates: 10.99 g

19. Tomato Artichoke Soup

Preparation Time: 5 minutes

Cooking Time: 35 minutes

Servings: 4

Ingredients:

- 1 can artichoke hearts, drained
- 1 can diced tomatoes, undrained
- 3 cups vegetable broth
- 1 small onion, chopped
- 2 cloves garlic, crushed
- 1 tbsp. pesto
- Black pepper, to taste

Directions:

1. Combine all ingredients in the slow cooker. Cover and cook on low within 8-10 hours or on high within 4-5 hours.
2. Blend the soup in batches then put it back to the slow cooker. Season with pepper and salt, then serve.

Nutrition: Calories: 1487 Protein: 3.98 g Fat: 167.42 g Carbohydrates: 8.2 g

20. Super Radish Avocado Salad

Preparation Time: 10 minutes

Cooking Time: 0 minutes

Servings: 2

Ingredients:

- 6 shredded carrots
- 6 ounces diced radishes
- 1 diced avocado
- 1/3 cup ponzu

Directions:

1. Place all together the ingredients in a serving bowl and toss. Enjoy!

Nutrition: Calories: 292 Protein: 7.42 g Fat: 18.29 g Carbohydrates: 29.59 g

21. Beauty School Ginger Cucumbers

Preparation Time: 10 minutes

Cooking Time: 0 minutes

Servings: 2

Ingredients:

- 1 sliced cucumber
- 3 tsp. rice wine vinegar
- 1 ½ tbsp. sugar
- 1 tsp. minced ginger

Directions:

1. Place all together the ingredients in a mixing bowl, and toss the ingredients well. Enjoy!

Nutrition: Calories: 10 Protein: 0.46 g Fat: 0.43 g Carbohydrates: 0.89 g

22. <u>Butternut Squash and Chickpea Curry</u>

Preparation Time: 20 minutes

Cooking Time: 6 hours

Servings: 8

Ingredients:

- 1 1/2 cups of shelled peas
- 1 1/2 cups of chickpeas, uncooked and rinsed
- 2 1/2 cups of diced butternut squash
- 12 ounces of chopped spinach
- 2 large tomatoes, diced
- 1 small white onion, peeled and chopped
- 1 teaspoon of minced garlic
- 1 teaspoon of salt
- 3 tablespoons of curry powder
- 14-ounce of coconut milk
- 3 cups of vegetable broth
- 1/4 cup of chopped cilantro

Directions:

1. Using a 6-quarts slow cooker, place all the ingredients into it except for the spinach and peas.
2. Cover the top, plug in the slow cooker; adjust the cooking time to 6 hours, and cook on the high heat setting or until the chickpeas get tender.

3. 30 minutes to ending your cooking, add the peas and spinach to the slow cooker and cook for the remaining 30 minutes.

4. Stir to check the sauce; if the sauce is runny, stir in a mixture of a 1 tbsp. Cornstarch mixed with 2 tbsp water. Serve with boiled rice.

Nutrition: Calories: 774 Protein: 3.71 g Fat: 83.25 g Carbohydrates: 12.64 g

SNACKS

23. Pesto Zucchini Noodles

Preparation Time: 15 minutes

Cooking Time: 0 minutes

Servings: 4

Ingredients:

- 4 little zucchini ends trimmed
- Cherry tomatoes
- 2 tsp fresh lemon juice
- 1/3 cup olive oil (best if extra-virgin)
- 2 cups packed basil leaves
- 2 cups garlic
- Salt and pepper to taste

Directions:

1. Spiral zucchini into noodles and set to the side. In a food processor, put the basil and garlic and chop. Slowly add olive oil while chopping. Then pulse blend it until thoroughly mixed.
2. In a big bowl, place the noodles and pour pesto sauce over the top.

3. Toss to combine. Garnish with tomatoes and serve and enjoy.

Nutrition: Calories: 173 Protein: 8.63 g Fat: 3.7 g Carbohydrates: 30.52 g

24. __Cabbage Slaw__

Preparation Time: 2 hours 5 minutes

Cooking Time: 0 minutes

Servings: 6

Ingredients:

- 1/8 tsp celery seed
- ¼ tsp salt
- 2 tbsp. of the following:
- Apple cider vinegar
- Sweetener of your choice
- ½ cup vegan mayo
- 4 cups coleslaw mix with red cabbage and carrots

Directions:

1. In a big mixing bowl, put and whisk together the celery seed, salt, apple cider vinegar, sweetener, and vegan mayo.
2. Add the coleslaw and stir until appropriately combined. Refrigerate while covered for a minimum of 2 hours or overnight if you're not in a hurry.

3. Garnish with tomatoes and serve and enjoy.

Nutrition: Calories: 136 Protein: 4.63 g Fat: 1.88 g Carbohydrates: 29.77 g

25. Avocado Sandwich

Preparation Time: 5 Minutes

Cooking Time: 5 Minutes

Servings: 2

Ingredients:

- 8 whole-wheat bread slices
- ½ oz. vegan butter
- 2 oz. little gem lettuce, cleaned and patted dry
- 1 oz. tofu cheese, sliced
- 1 avocado, pitted, peeled, and sliced
- 1 small cucumber, sliced into 4 rings
- Freshly chopped parsley to garnish

Directions:

1. Arrange the 4 bread slices on a flat surface and smear the vegan butter on one end each. Place a lettuce leaf on each and arrange some tofu cheese on top. Top with the avocado and cucumber slices.
2. Garnish the sandwiches with a little parsley, cover with the remaining bread slices, and serve immediately.

Nutrition: Calories: 380 Fat: 21g Carbs: 44g Protein: 9.0g

26. <u>Tacos</u>

Preparation Time: 10 Minutes

Cooking Time: 30 Minutes

Servings: 4

Ingredients:

- 6 Taco Shells
- For the slaw:
- 1 cup Red Cabbage, shredded
- 3 Scallions, chopped
- 1 cup Green Cabbage, shredded
- 1 cup Carrots, sliced
- For the dressing:
- 1 tbsp. Sriracha
- ¼ cup Apple Cider Vinegar
- ¼ tsp. Salt
- 2 tbsp. Sesame Oil
- 1 tbsp. Dijon Mustard
- 1 tbsp. Lime Juice
- ½ tbsp. Tamari
- 1 tbsp. Maple Syrup
- ¼ tsp. Salt

Directions:

1. For the dressing, put and whisk all the ingredients in a small bowl until mixed well. Next, combine the slaw ingredients in another bowl and toss well.

2. Finally, take a taco shell and place the slaw in it. Serve and enjoy.

Nutrition: Calories: 216 Protein: 10g Carbohydrates: 15g Fat: 13g

VEGETABLES

27. Crusty Grilled Corn

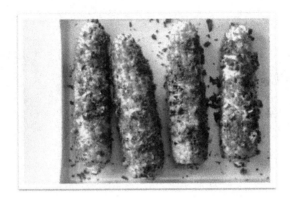

Preparation Time: 10 minutes

Cooking Time: 15 minutes

Servings: 4

Ingredients:

- 2 corn cobs
- 1/3 cup Vegenaise
- 1 small handful cilantro
- ½ cup breadcrumbs
- 1 teaspoon lemon juice

Directions:

1. Preheat the gas grill on high heat.

2. Add corn grill to the grill and continue grilling until it turns golden-brown on all sides.
3. Mix the Vegenaise, cilantro, breadcrumbs, and lemon juice in a bowl.
4. Add grilled corn cobs to the crumb's mixture.
5. Toss well then serve.

Nutrition: Calories: 253 Total Fat: 13g Protein: 31g Total Carbs: 3g Fiber: 0g Net Carbs: 3g

28. **Grilled Carrots with Chickpea Salad**

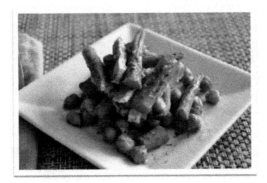

Preparation Time: 10 minutes

Cooking Time: 10 minutes

Servings: 8

Ingredients:

- Carrots
- 8 large carrots
- 1 tablespoon oil
- 1 ½ teaspoon salt
- 1 teaspoon dried oregano
- 1 teaspoon dried thyme
- 2 teaspoon paprika powder
- 1 ½ tablespoon soy sauce
- ½ cup of water
- Chickpea Salad
- 14 oz canned chickpeas
- 3 medium pickles

- 1 small onion
- A big handful of lettuce
- 1 teaspoon apple cider vinegar
- ½ teaspoon dried oregano
- ½ teaspoon salt
- Ground black pepper, to taste
- ½ cup vegan cream

Directions:

1. Toss the carrots with all of its ingredients in a bowl.
2. Thread one carrot on a stick and place it on a plate.
3. Preheat the grill over high heat.
4. Grill the carrots for 2 minutes per side on the grill.
5. Toss the ingredients for the salad in a large salad bowl.
6. Slice grilled carrots and add them on top of the salad.
7. Serve fresh.

Nutrition: Calories: 661 Total Fat: 68g Carbs: 17g Net Carbs: 7g Fiber: 2g Protein: 4g

29. <u>**Grilled Avocado Guacamole**</u>

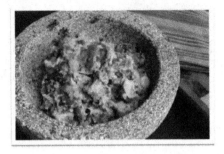

Preparation Time: 10 minutes

Cooking Time: 20 minutes

Servings: 4

Ingredients:

- ½ teaspoon olive oil
- 1 lime, halved
- ½ onion, halved
- 1 serrano chile, halved, stemmed, and seeded
- 3 Haas avocados, skin on
- 2–3 tablespoons fresh cilantro, chopped
- ½ teaspoon smoked salt

Directions:

1. Preheat the grill over medium heat.
2. Brush the grilling grates with olive oil and place chile, onion, and lime on it.
3. Grill the onion for 10 minutes, chile for 5 minutes, and lime for 2 minutes.

4. Transfer the veggies to a large bowl.
5. Now cut the avocados in half and grill them for 5 minutes.
6. Mash the flesh of the grilled avocado in a bowl.
7. Chop the other grilled veggies and add them to the avocado mash.
8. Stir in remaining ingredients and mix well.
9. Serve.

Nutrition: Calories: 165 Total Fat: 17g Carbs: 4g Net Carbs: 2g Fiber: 1g Protein: 1g

SALAD

30. Jicama and Spinach Salad Recipe

Preparation Time: 10 minutes

Cooking Time: 20 minutes

Servings: 4

Ingredients:

- Salad:
- 10 oz baby spinach, washed and dried
- Grape or cherry tomatoes, cut in half
- 1 jicama, washed, peeled, and cut in strips
- Green or Kalamata olives, chopped
- 8 tsp walnuts, chopped
- 1 tsp raw or roasted sunflower seeds
- Maple Mustard Dressing
- **Dressing:**
- 1 heaping tbsp Dijon mustard
- Dash cayenne pepper
- 2 tbsp maple syrup
- 2 garlic cloves, minced
- 1 to 2 tbsp water

- ¼ tsp sea salt
- For the salad:

Directions:

1. Divide the baby spinach onto 4 salad plates. Top each serving with ¼ of the jicama, ¼ of the chopped olives, and 4 tomatoes. Sprinkle 1 tsp of the sunflower seeds and 2 tsp of the walnuts.

   For the dressing:

2. In a small mixing bowl, whisk all the ingredients together until emulsified. Check the taste and add more maple syrup for sweetness.

3. Drizzle 1½ tbsp of the dressing over each salad and serve.

Nutrition: Calories: 196 Fat: 2 g Protein: 7 g Carbs: 28 g Fiber: 12g

31. <u>High-Protein Salad</u>

Preparation Time: 5 minutes

Cooking Time: 5 minutes

Servings: 4

Ingredients:

- Salad:
- 1 15-oz can green kidney beans
- 2 4 tbsp capers
- 3 4 handfuls arugula
- 4 15-oz can lentils
  Dressing:
- 5 1 tbsp caper brine
- 6 1 tbsp tamari
- 7 1 tbsp balsamic vinegar
- 8 2 tbsp peanut butter
- 9 2 tbsp hot sauce
- 10 1 tbsp tahini

Directions:

1. For the dressing:
2. In a bowl, whisk together all the ingredients until they come together to form a smooth dressing.
3. For the salad:

4. Mix the beans, arugula, capers, and lentils. Top with the dressing and serve.

Nutrition: Calories: 205 Fat: 2 g Protein: 13 g Carbs: 31 g Fiber: 17g

GRAINS

32. **Noodle and Rice Pilaf**

Preparation Time: 5 minutes

Cooking Time: 33 to 44 minutes

Servings: 6 to 8

Ingredients:

- 1 cup whole-wheat noodles, broken into 1/8-inch pieces
- 2 cups long-grain brown rice
- 6½ cups low-sodium vegetable broth
- 1 teaspoon ground cumin
- ½ teaspoon dried oregano

Directions:

1. Combine the noodles and rice in a saucepan over medium heat and cook for 3 to 4 minutes, or until they begin to smell toasted.
2. Stir in the vegetable broth, cumin and oregano. Bring to a boil. Reduce the heat to medium-low. Cover and cook for 30 to 40 minutes, or until all water is absorbed.

Nutrition: calories: 287 fat: 2.5g carbs: 58.1g protein: 7.9gfiber: 5.0g

33. <u>Easy Millet Loaf</u>

Preparation Time: 5 minutes

Cooking Time: 1 hour 15 minutes

Servings: 4

Ingredients:

- 1¼ cups millet
- 4 cups unsweetened tomato juice
- 1 medium onion, chopped
- 1 to 2 cloves garlic
- ½ teaspoon dried sage
- ½ teaspoon dried basil
- ½ teaspoon poultry seasoning

Directions:

1. Preheat the oven to 350°F (180°C).
2. Place the millet in a large bowl.
3. Place the remaining ingredients in a blender and pulse until smooth. Add to the bowl with the millet and mix well.
4. Pour the mixture into a shallow casserole dish. Cover and bake in the oven for 1¼ hours, or until set.

5. Serve warm.

Nutrition: calories: 315 fat: 3.4g carbs: 61.6g protein: 10.2g fiber: 9.6g

LEGUMES

34. Classic Italian Minestrone

Preparation Time: 10 minutes

Cooking Time: 10 minutes

Servings: 4

Ingredients:

- 2 tablespoons olive oil
- 1 large onion, diced
- 2 carrots, sliced
- 4 cloves garlic, minced
- 1 cup elbow pasta
- 5 cups vegetable broth
- 1 (15-ounce) can white beans, drained
- 1 large zucchini, diced
- 1 (28-ounce) can tomatoes, crushed
- 1 tablespoon fresh oregano leaves, chopped
- 1 tablespoon fresh basil leaves, chopped
- 1 tablespoon fresh Italian parsley, chopped

Directions

1. In a Dutch oven, heat the olive oil until sizzling. Now, sauté the onion and carrots until they've softened.

2. Add in the garlic, uncooked pasta and broth; let it simmer for about 15 minutes.

3. Stir in the beans, zucchini, tomatoes and herbs. Continue to cook, covered, for about 10 minutes until everything is thoroughly cooked.

4. Garnish with some extra herbs, if desired. Bon appétit!

Nutrition: Calories: 305; Fat: 8.6g; Carbs: 45.1g; Protein: 14.2g

35. Green Lentil Stew with Collard Greens

Preparation Time: 10 minutes

Cooking Time: 10 minutes

Servings: 4

Ingredients:

- 2 tablespoons olive oil
- 1 onion, chopped
- 2 sweet potatoes, peeled and diced
- 1 bell pepper, chopped
- 2 carrots, chopped
- 1 parsnip, chopped
- 1 celery, chopped
- 2 cloves garlic
- 1 ½ cups green lentils
- 1 tablespoon Italian herb mix
- 1 cup tomato sauce
- 5 cups vegetable broth
- 1 cup frozen corn
- 1 cup collard greens, torn into pieces

Directions

1. In a Dutch oven, heat the olive oil until sizzling. Now, sauté the onion, sweet potatoes, bell pepper, carrots, parsnip and celery until they've softened.

2. Add in the garlic and continue sautéing an additional 30 seconds.
3. Now, add in the green lentils, Italian herb mix, tomato sauce and vegetable broth; let it simmer for about 20 minutes until everything is thoroughly cooked.
4. Add in the frozen corn and collard greens; cover and let it simmer for 5 minutes more. Bon appétit!

Nutrition: Calories: 415; Fat: 6.6g; Carbs: 71g; Protein: 18.4g

36. <u>Chickpea Garden Vegetable Medley</u>

Preparation Time: 10 minutes

Cooking Time: 10 minutes

Servings: 4

Ingredients:

- 2 tablespoons olive oil
- 1 onion, finely chopped
- 1 bell pepper, chopped
- 1 fennel bulb, chopped
- 3 cloves garlic, minced
- 2 ripe tomatoes, pureed
- 2 tablespoons fresh parsley, roughly chopped
- 2 tablespoons fresh basil, roughly chopped
- 2 tablespoons fresh coriander, roughly chopped
- 2 cups vegetable broth
- 14 ounces canned chickpeas, drained
- Kosher salt and ground black pepper, to taste
- 1/2 teaspoon cayenne pepper
- 1 teaspoon paprika
- 1 avocado, peeled and sliced

Directions

1. In a heavy-bottomed pot, heat the olive oil over medium heat. Once hot, sauté the onion, bell pepper and fennel bulb for about 4 minutes.
2. Sauté the garlic for about 1 minute or until aromatic.
3. Add in the tomatoes, fresh herbs, broth, chickpeas, salt, black pepper, cayenne pepper and paprika. Let it simmer, stirring occasionally, for about 20 minutes or until cooked through.
4. Taste and adjust the seasonings. Serve garnished with the slices of the fresh avocado. Bon appétit!

Nutrition: Calories: 369; Fat: 18.1g; Carbs: 43.5g; Protein: 13.2g

BREAD & PIZZA

37. Incredible Artichoke and Olives Pizza

Preparation time: 20 minutes

Cooking time: 1 hour 50 minutes

Servings: 6

Ingredients:

- 12 inch of frozen whole-wheat pizza crust, thawed
- 1 mushroom, sliced
- 1/2 cup of sliced char-grilled artichokes
- 1 small green bell pepper, cored and sliced
- 2 medium-sized tomatoes, sliced
- 2 tablespoons of sliced black olives
- 1/2 teaspoon of garlic powder
- 1 teaspoon of salt, divided
- 1/2 teaspoon of dried oregano
- 2 tablespoons of nutritional yeast
- 2-ounce cashews
- 2 teaspoons of lemon juice
- 3 tablespoon of olive oil, divided
- 8-ounce of tomato paste

- 4 fluid ounces of water

Directions:

1. Place the cashews in a food processor; add the garlic powder, 1/2 teaspoon of salt, yeast, 2 tablespoons of oil, lemon juice, and water.
2. Mash it until it gets smooth and creamy, but add some water if need be.
3. Grease a 4 to 6 quarts slow cooker with a non-stick cooking spray and insert the pizza crust into it.
4. Press the dough in bottom and spread the tomato paste on top of it.
5. Sprinkle it with garlic powder, oregano and top it with the prepared cashew mixture.
6. Spray it with the mushrooms, bell peppers, tomato, artichoke slices, olives and then with the remaining olive oil.
7. Sprinkle it with the oregano, the remaining salt and cover it with the lid.
8. Plug in the slow cooker and let it cook for 1 to 1 1/2 hours at the low heat setting or until the crust turns golden brown.

9. When done, transfer the pizza to the cutting board, let it rest for 10 minutes and slice to serve.

Nutrition: Calories: 212 Cal, Carbohydrates: 39g, Protein: 16g, Fats: 5g, Fiber: 5g.

38. **<u>Mushroom and Peppers Pizza</u>**

Preparation time: 20 minutes

Cooking time: 2 hours

Servings: 6

Ingredients:

- 12 inch of frozen whole-wheat pizza crust, thawed
- 1/2 cup of chopped red bell pepper
- 1/2 cup of chopped green bell pepper
- 1/2 cup of chopped orange bell pepper
- 3/4 cup of chopped button mushrooms
- 1 small red onion, peeled and chopped
- 1 teaspoon of garlic powder, divided
- 1 teaspoon of salt, divided
- 1/2 teaspoon of coconut sugar
- 1/2 teaspoon of red pepper flakes
- 1 teaspoon of dried basil, divided
- 1 1/2 teaspoon of dried oregano, divided
- 1 tablespoon of olive oil
- 6-ounce of tomato paste
- 1/2 cup of vegan Parmesan cheese

Directions:

1. Place a large non-stick skillet pan over an average heat, add the oil and let it heat.

2. Add the onion, bell peppers and cook for 10 minutes or until it gets soft and lightly charred. Then add the mushroom, cook it for 3 minutes and set the pan aside until it is needed.

3. Pour the tomato sauce, sugar, 1/2 teaspoon of the garlic powder, salt, basil, oregano, into a bowl and stir properly.

4. Grease a 4 to 6 quarts slow cooker with a non-stick cooking spray and insert the pizza crust into it.

5. Press the dough in bottom and spread the already prepared tomato sauce on top of it. Sprinkle it with the Parmesan cheese and top it with the cooked vegetable mixture.

6. Cover it with the lid, plug in the slow cooker and let it cook for 1 to 1 1/2 hours at the low heat setting or until the crust turns golden brown.

7. When done, transfer the pizza to a cutting board, sprinkle it with the remaining oregano, basil, then let it rest for 10 minutes and then slice to serve.

Nutrition: Calories: 188 Cal, Carbohydrates: 27g, Protein: 5g, Fats: 5g, Fiber: 3g.

SOUP AND STEW

39. Pesto Pea Soup

Preparation Time: 10 Minutes

Cooking Time: 20 Minutes

Servings: 4

Ingredients:

- 2 cups Water
- 8 oz. Tortellini
- ¼ cup Pesto
- 1 Onion, small & finely chopped
- 1 lb. Peas, frozen
- 1 Carrot, medium & finely chopped
- 1 ¾ cup Vegetable Broth, less sodium
- 1 Celery Rib, medium & finely chopped

Directions:

1. To start with, boil the water in a large pot over a medium-high heat.
2. Next, stir in the tortellini to the pot and cook it following the packet's instructions.
3. In the meantime, cook the onion, celery, and carrot in a deep saucepan along with the water and broth.

4. Cook the celery-onion mixture for 6 minutes or until softened.
5. Now, spoon in the peas and allow it to simmer while keeping it uncovered.
6. Cook the peas for few minutes or until they are bright green and soft.
7. Then, spoon in the pesto to the pea's mixture. Combine well.
8. Pour the mixture into a high-speed blender and blend for 2 to 3 minutes or until you get a rich, smooth soup.
9. Return the soup to the pan. Spoon in the cooked tortellini.
10. Finally, pour into a serving bowl and top with more cooked peas if desired.
11. Tip: If desired, you can season it with Maldon salt at the end.

Nutrition: Calories 100 Fat 0 g Protein 0 g Carbohydrates 0 g

40. Tofu and Mushroom Soup

Preparation Time: 15 Minutes

Cooking Time: 10 Minutes

Servings: 4

Ingredients:

- 2 tbsp olive oil
- 1 garlic clove, minced
- 1 large yellow onion, finely chopped
- 1 tsp freshly grated ginger
- 1 cup vegetable stock
- 2 small potatoes, peeled and chopped
- ¼ tsp salt
- ¼ tsp black pepper
- 2 (14 oz) silken tofu, drained and rinsed
- 2/3 cup baby Bella mushrooms, sliced
- 1 tbsp chopped fresh oregano
- 2 tbsp chopped fresh parsley to garnish

Directions:

1. Heat the olive oil in a medium pot over medium heat and sauté the garlic, onion, and ginger until soft and fragrant.
2. Pour in the vegetable stock, potatoes, salt, and black pepper. Cook until the potatoes soften, 12 minutes.

3. Stir in the tofu and using an immersion blender, puree the ingredients until smooth.
4. Mix in the mushrooms and simmer with the pot covered until the mushrooms warm up while occasionally stirring to ensure that the tofu doesn't curdle, 7 minutes.
5. Stir oregano, and dish the soup.
6. Garnish with the parsley and serve warm.

Nutrition: Calories 310 Fat 10 g Protein 40.0 g Carbohydrates 0 g

SAUCES, DRESSINGS & DIP

41.   Pumpkin Spice Spread

Preparation Time: 10 minutes

Cooking Time: 10 minutes

Servings: 4

Ingredients:

- 1 package (8 oz.) fat-free cream cheese
- 1/2 cup canned pumpkin
- Sugar substitute equivalent to 1/2 cup sugar
- 1 teaspoon ground cinnamon
- 1 teaspoon vanilla extract
- 1 teaspoon maple flavoring
- 1/2 teaspoon pumpkin pie spice
- 1/2 teaspoon ground nutmeg
- 1 carton (8 oz.) frozen reduced-fat whipped topping, thawed

Directions:

1. Mix well together sugar substitute, pumpkin, and cream cheese in a big bowl. Beat in nutmeg, pumpkin pie spice, maple flavoring, vanilla, and cinnamon.

2. Fold in whipped topping and chill until serving.

Nutrition: calories 177 fat 6 carbs 21 protein 11

42. **Maple Bagel Spread**

Preparation Time: 10 minutes

Cooking Time: 10 minutes

Servings: 1

Ingredients:

- cream cheese
- maple syrup
- cinnamon
- walnuts

Directions:

1. Beat the cinnamon, syrup, and cream cheese in a big bowl until it becomes smooth, then mix in walnuts.
2. Let it chill until ready to serve. Serve it with bagels.

Nutrition: calories 586 fat 7 carbs 23 protein 4

APPETIZER

43. White Beans and Avocado Toast

Preparation Time: 5 minutes

Cooking Time: 1 minutes

Servings: 1

Ingredients:

1 slice Whole-wheat bread

¼ Avocado

½ cup Canned white beans, rinsed and drained

Kosher salt, as per taste

Ground pepper, as per taste

Crushed red pepper

Directions:

Start by taking a toaster and placing the whole-wheat bread in it to toast. Once done, remove and keep aside. Take a small bowl and mash to avocado.

Take the canned white beans and thoroughly rinse and drain them. Place the toast on a plate and top it with mashed avocado.

Place the white beans on top as well. Nicely season with pepper, salt and red pepper. Serve.

Nutrition: Calories: 307 Carbs: 37g Fat: 6g Protein: 14g

44. Fresh Edamame Pods with Aleppo Pepper

Preparation Time: 0 minutes

Cooking Time: 5 minutes

Servings: 1

Ingredients

½ cup Edamame (in pods)

1/8 tsp Aleppo pepper

Directions:

Start by taking a steamer and place it over high flame. Fill it with water and let it come to a boil.

Place the edamame pods in the steamer and steam for about 5 minutes. The pods should be crisp and tender. Transfer into a serving platter and sprinkle with Aleppo pepper.

Nutrition: Calories: 124 Carbs: 12g Fat: 4g Protein: 10g

45. <u>Toast with Cannellini Beans and Pesto</u>

Preparation Time: 5 minutes

Cooking Time: 0 minutes

Servings: 1

Ingredients:

1 slice Whole-wheat bread (toasted)

1/3 cup Canned cannellini beans (no-salt added)

1 pinch Garlic powder

½ teaspoon Basil pesto

2 tablespoons Tomato (chopped)

Directions:

Start by rinsing and draining the canned cannellini beans. Keep aside. Take the toasted slice and place it on a plate.

Take a small mixing bowl and add in the beans, tomatoes and garlic powder. Mix well. Place the prepared beans and tomatoes mixture on the toast and top with pesto. Serve.

Nutrition: Calories: 366 Carbs: 49g Fat: 12g Protein: 21g

DESSERTS

46. <u>Walnut Zucchini Bread</u>

Preparation time: 15 minutes

Cooking time: 60 minutes

Servings: 9

Ingredients:

- Nonstick cooking spray
- 2 cups almond flour
- ½ teaspoon ground cinnamon
- 1 teaspoon baking soda
- 2 large organic eggs
- 1/3 cup grass-fed butter, at room temperature
- ½ cup erythritol, granulated
- 1½ cups grated and squeezed dry zucchini
- 1/3 cup sugar-free chocolate chips

Directions:

1. Preheat the oven to 350°F. Grease a bread loaf pan with cooking spray. In a medium bowl, sift together the almond flour, cinnamon, and baking soda. Set aside.

2. Beat the eggs, butter, and erythritol in the bowl of a stand mixer until combined, 1 to 2 minutes. Stir in the zucchini.

3. Put the flour batter to the egg batter. Blend until only just combined. Mix in the chocolate chips.

4. Put the batter into your loaf pan and cook for 1 hour, or until a toothpick inserted in the middle comes out clean.

Nutrition: Calories: 175 Fat: 15g Protein: 5g Carbs: 5g

47. <u>Chocolate Peanut Butter Cups</u>

Preparation time: 20 minutes

Cooking time: 0 minutes

Servings: 6

Ingredients:

For the chocolate layer:

- Nonstick cooking spray
- 2 tablespoons coconut oil, melted
- 4 tablespoons creamy natural peanut butter
- 2 tablespoons unsweetened cocoa powder
- 4 or 5 drops liquid stevia
- For the peanut butter layer:
- 2 tablespoons coconut oil, melted
- 4 tablespoons natural peanut butter
- ¼ teaspoon vanilla extract
- 4 or 5 drops liquid stevia

Directions:

1. For the chocolate layer, spray the cups of a 12-cup mini muffin pan with cooking spray. Whisk all the fixings in a small bowl until well combined.
2. Fill the bottom of each muffin cup with about 2 teaspoons of the mixture. Place in the freezer to set for about 8 minutes.

3. For the peanut butter layer, while the chocolate layer is freezing, in a small bowl, combine all the ingredients for the peanut butter layer and mix well.

4. To assemble the cups, remove the muffin tin from the freezer and top each chocolate layer with 2 teaspoons of peanut butter mixture.

5. Put the muffin tin back in your freezer and freeze for a further 8 minutes. Use a butter knife to remove the cups from the tin and place them in a resealable plastic freezer bag. Store in the freezer.

Nutrition: Calories: 224 Fat: 20g Protein: 5g Carbs: 5g

48. Keto-Friendly Key Lime Pie

Preparation time: 4 hours & 15 minutes

Cooking time: 12 minutes

Servings: 6

Ingredients:

For the crust:

- Nonstick cooking spray
- 2 tablespoons coconut oil, melted
- 1 cup almond flour
- 1 tablespoon coconut flour
- 1 egg
- 1/8 teaspoon salt
- For the filling:
- 2 tablespoons coconut flour
- 2 (14-ounce) cans coconut cream
- 1/3 cup freshly squeezed lime juice
- Zest of 2 limes
- For the topping:
- 2 cups heavy cream, whipped
- 2 teaspoons erythritol, for the whipped cream

Directions:

1. Preheat the oven to 350°F. Oiled a 9-inch pie plate with cooking spray. In the bowl of a food processor or a

high-speed blender, combine the coconut oil, almond flour, coconut flour, egg, and salt. Pulse until crumbly.

2. Pour the mixture into the prepared pie plate and use a fork to press the crust down evenly. Bake for about 12 minutes, then set aside to cool for 10 minutes.

3. While the crust is cooling, in a medium bowl, use a hand mixer to mix together the coconut flour, coconut cream, lime juice, and lime zest for 1 to 2 minutes.

4. Pour the filling into the cooled crust and cover with plastic wrap. Refrigerate within at least 4 hours to set. Remove, slice, and top with the whipped cream.

Nutrition: Calories: 814 Fat: 83g Protein: 10g Carbs: 17g

SMOOTHIES AND JUICES

49. Kiwi and Strawberry Smoothie

Preparation Time: 5 minutes

Cooking Time: 0 minutes

Servings: 3

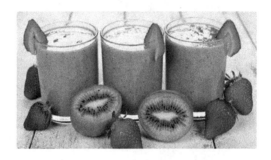

Ingredients:

- 1 kiwi, peeled
- 5 medium strawberries
- ½ frozen banana
- 1 cup unsweetened almond milk
- 2 tablespoons hemp seeds
- 2 tablespoons peanut butter
- 1 to 2 teaspoons maple syrup
- ½ cup spinach leaves
- Handful broccoli sprouts

Directions:

1. Put all the ingredients in a food processor, then blitz until creamy and smooth.
2. Serve immediately or chill in the refrigerator for an hour before serving.

Nutrition: calories: 562 fat: 28.6g carbs: 63.6g fiber: 15.1g protein: 23.3g